Natural Healing for a Lifestyle Change

Eunice Clarke

© 2016 Eunice Clarke
All Rights Reserved
ISBN-13: 978-1539897798
ISBN-10: 1539897796

This Manual is dedicated to those persons who seriously choose to make a commitment to their health and desire some assistance for a lifestyle change to RENEW, RESTORE, and REJUVENATE their bodies to achieve maximum health benefits.

DISCLAIMER

This Manual is not to be used to diagnose. It is not a claim to mitigate disease either. You are encouraged to follow the recommendations of your health care provider.

Rather, this manual is meant for information purposes to educate the reader on prevention, healthy choices, and alternative approaches which have proven effective in alleviating ailments and in creating youth and vitality.

All information presented in this manual is meant to educate and enlighten the reader - it is not meant to be used in place of medical procedure or as a substitute for medical care and should not be used as such.

Rather, this information is to provide awareness that expands logical thinking. As a result, the reader may view the matter from a much broader perspective.

HEALING JOURNEY

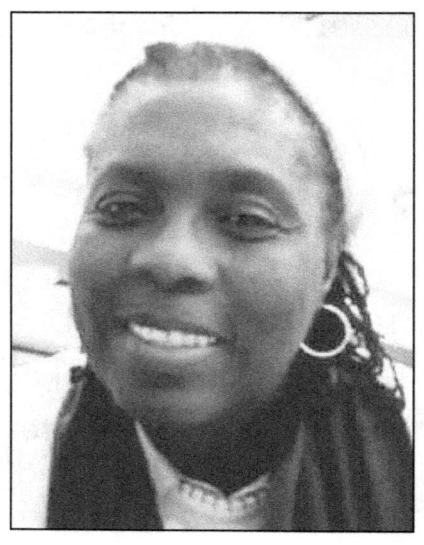

What you are about to read in this manual you are already familiar with; now, you are just being reminded of a few important things. This is how I view the material contents presented herein on these pages.

I feel deeply grateful to be writing this manual and presenting the contents that hopefully will guide you to a lifestyle change. For about half my life, I have been directly engaged in helping people learn to feel better and achieve peace and comfort in their lives.

During this time, I have been a consumer of natural healing remedies, treatment modalities and learning to apply effective methods and techniques. I have reaped many benefits in every imaginable way from many processes and proven ideas that I share in this manual.

I am presenting you with what I am familiar, which is some of my knowledge about cleansing and detoxifying as part of my personal journey. This is the culmination of my life's dream. Most of the contents are taken from experiences of my personal journey during my own quest to find meaning to my healing and restoration.

I believed and still do, that God's plan for man, is to be healthy in body, mind, and spirit. I do sincerely believe that when I change my thinking, I will change my world for a more positive style of living. Then my World will be the GARDEN OF EDEN.

However, I must be a responsible keeper of this body temple, keeping it fit and whole. Hopefully, some thoughts here can help free you from the impediment of thinking "sickness" instead of health and wellness. This will move you from "victim to victor."

Knowing the power that you have within your own being, you can achieve whatever you desire. It is also beneficial to put a price value on yourself, either a 50 cent value or a 50-billion-dollar value. Which one fits you? The whole meaning to this is to think of yourself as most valuable.

You are worthy of the highest and best - a special part of GOD's creative plan. This Manual is therefore intended as a guide to help you start the process of your own journey. However, you are encouraged to research further and go beyond this preliminary work for yourself. Cleanse and detoxify from inside out and discover your feeling of love, joy and happiness that testifies to everyone and everything around.

With Love,

Eunice M. Clarke
Holistic Nurse and Christian Counselor
Founder and Director of the Holistic Institute of Healing
Bullet Tree Falls, Belize

> To quote the great philosopher, Hippocrates, "Let your food be your medicine and your medicine be your food." As a result, that which we put into the body can purify, cleanse and rejuvenate the organs and cells of

The intestinal tract and digestive system serve as a central point for all the organs and cells of the body. They are totally dependent on a well-functioning system. According to much research, it is said that 95% of disease starts in the colon and spreads to other parts of the body.

Statistical information shows, in recent years, there has been marked increase in diseases of the Gastrointestinal Tract including the colon and related organs. Research figures are teaming with reports on health problems, such as obesity, diabetes, hypertension and other ailments are directly related to poor nutritional health both in adults and children. Much argument is that many illnesses can be prevented if individuals will have guidance and educational instructions. That is all the more reason for presenting this information.

> Think about this! You clean out your car, you clean out your home, is it not more beneficial to your well-being to clean out yourself from the inside out? KEEP THE BODY AS A LIVING TEMPLE, WHERE THE SPIRIT DWELLS.

INTRODUCTION

There are many volumes written that give directions on the subject of good health and how to achieve balance in the body systems. First, we will discuss Ayurvedic treatment. Ayurvedic herbal treatment modality has its origin in India and is used here in this document to address issues on restoring health in the gastrointestinal system.

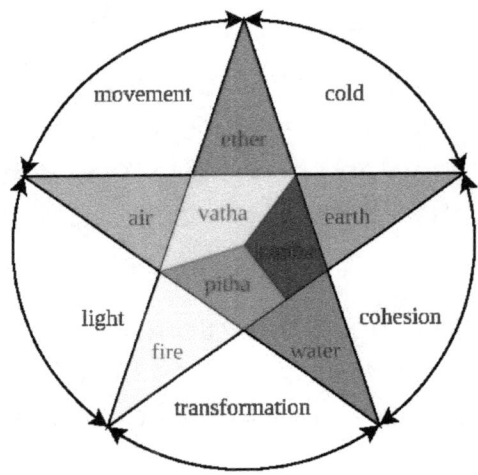

Ayurveda addresses issues on rekindling the digestive fire and achieving health from the inside out. The philosophy states that the root cause of disease is the malfunctioning of the body's metabolic system's main fire of digestion, called Agni.

Agni is the action of the metabolic process that breaks down and transforms food to be used by the body system as nutrients. Its major premise is that if this essential part of the digestion is functioning effectively then the whole body will be nourished and supported. Consequently, the whole will be nourished, energized, vibrant and healthy.

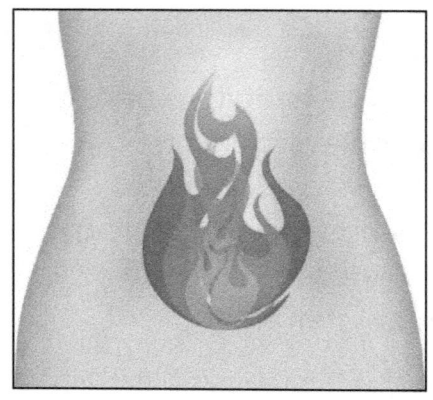
The digestive fire or Agni is likened to the fire in a wood-burning stove or fire-heart. The black soot that emits from the burning is called Ama which causes a buildup that is thick, black, and tarry. The more efficiently the wood burns in the stove, the less soot it created.

Similarly, there is a buildup of Ama or toxic waste started in the GI System accumulates in many of the organs of the body. Agni energizes the body, while Ama is the accumulation in the tissues and organs causing it to malfunction.

Agni is hot, dry, light, clear, and aromatic wherein Ama is wet, cold, heavy, sticky, and bad smelling. Treatment focuses on increasing Agni, the Digestive Fire, and Ama will come into balance.

The root cause of all disease is an accumulation of toxic buildup resulting from improper metabolism and functioning of the digestive system. When undigested food material accumulates in the bowel it becomes sour, foul smelling, and appears as a sticky mucoid substance.

This is Ama, its mucus clogs the blood vessels, capillaries, and other vital organs with mucus. Eventually, these toxic products weaken parts of the body, create blockages, stagnation, and a general decrease in function of the immune system. Finally, this toxicity manifests in disease states such as heart disease, cancer and immune system breakdown.

How does Ama form and what are signs that one's Agni and Ama are out of balance?

1. When a person eats mucous forming foods or poor food combinations, Ama is increased and Agni is decreased. This causes increased weight and many of the already mentioned symptoms of toxic buildup.

2. Whitish-yellowish coating on the tongue is a clear indication of Ama toxicity in the digestive system.

3. Thin and emaciated. Symptoms of high Agni because the digestive process burns away the normal digestive nutrients too fast.

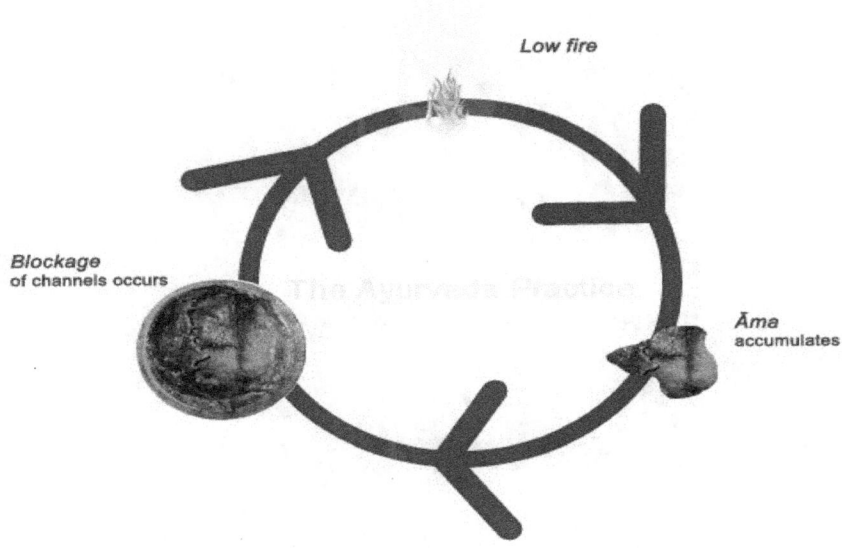

STICK-TO-IT-NESS, commits to a wholesome life-style. Here are a few pointers and quotes that may contribute to your enhancement and helping you to STICK- TO-IT, and embrace a wholesome lifestyle. So what is missing now? YOUR COMMITMENT!

What are some common symptoms of toxic buildup? -bad breath, loss of appetite, indigestion, coated tongue, body odor, low energy, weight gain, feeling sluggish, decreased energy, constipation, depression, dull pulse beat, obstruction of body channels, to name a few.

12

HUGGING

The basic essentials of life are air, water, food, clothing, shelter, and hugging.

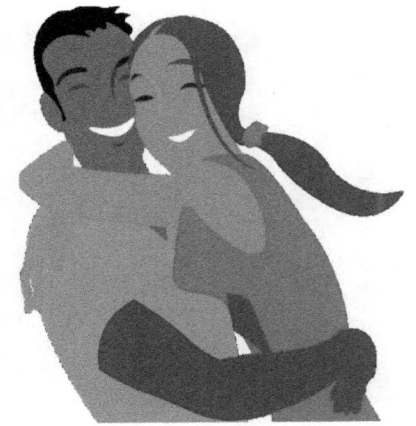

Hugging is **natural:**

- Organic
- Naturally Sweet
- No pesticides
- No preservatives
- No Artificial Ingredients
- 100% Wholesome

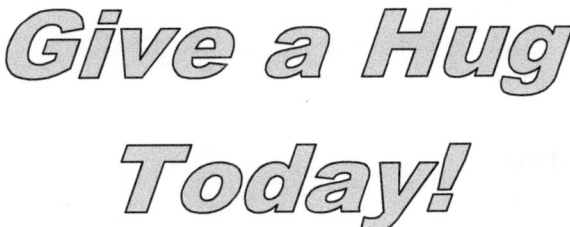

Hugging is **healthy**:

- It helps the body's immune system
- It keeps you healthier
- Cures depression
- It reduces stress
- It induces sleep
- It's invigorating
- It's rejuvenating
- It has no unpleasant side effects
- Hugging is nothing less than a miracle drug

Hugging is **practically perfect**:

- No moveable parts
- No batteries to wear out
- No periodic checkups
- Low energy consumption
- High energy yield
- Inflation proof
- Not flattening
- No monthly payments
- No insurance requirements
- No nicotine
- Fully refundable

Best people, places, and times to hug:

Anyone - any place - any time There's a hug to say I love you. There's a hug to say goodbye. There's a hug to say, how are you? And a hug to say we tried! There's a hug to bond a friendship and a hug when the day is through... But the hug I love in all the world is the hug I get from you! Hugs are free,

maybe that is why so many people take them for granted. If hugs cost a lot of money, people would probably knock themselves out to make money to buy hugs. Even though hugs are free, hugs aren't worth anything if they aren't used... and a hug not used is a hug lost forever.

Author: unknown

LOVE

Love is a concern for the welfare of others. Love is a feeling we have towards another which is like the feeling we have for ourselves. Love is our desire for happiness of other persons. Love is essential to our experience in the psychic realm and use of its powers, because in the unobstructed universe we are one with all spiritual beings, working together for common goals. As spirit beings we must love ourselves, or we will use our powers to destroy parts of ourselves which would cause sorrow to ourselves.

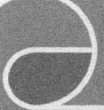

If man is to speak in the tongues of men and of angels, but have not love, he is as noisy gong or a clanging cymbal.

And if man has prophetic powers, and understand all mysteries and all knowledge. And if he has not all faith so as to remove mountains, but has not love, he is nothing. And if I deliver my body to be burned but have not love, I gain nothing.

Love is patient and kind. Love is not jealous or boastful; it is not arrogant or rude. Love does not insist on its own way; it is not irritable or resentful; it does not rejoice at wrong, but rejoices in the right. Love bears all things, hopes all things, endures all things.

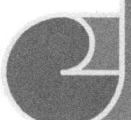

1 Corinthians. Chapter 13

"Take care to get what you like or you will end up having to like what you get. It is your words that speak loudly of your intentions and actions speak louder than words. Commitment is making the time when there is none. It is the stuff character is made of: The power to change the face of things. It is the daily triumph of integrity over skepticism."

- George Bernard Shaw

Commitment is what transforms a promise into reality it is the words that speak boldly of your intentions and your actions which speak louder than words. It is making the time when there is none, coming through time after time, year after year. Commitment is the stuff character is made of; the power to change the face of things. It is the daily triumph of integrity over skepticism.

- Author Unknown

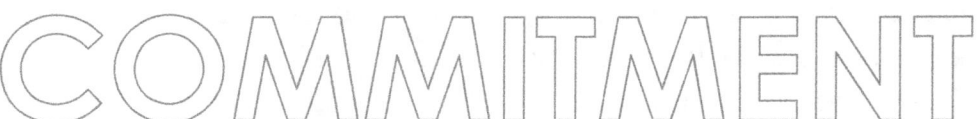

CLEANSE AND DETOXIFY YOUR BODY

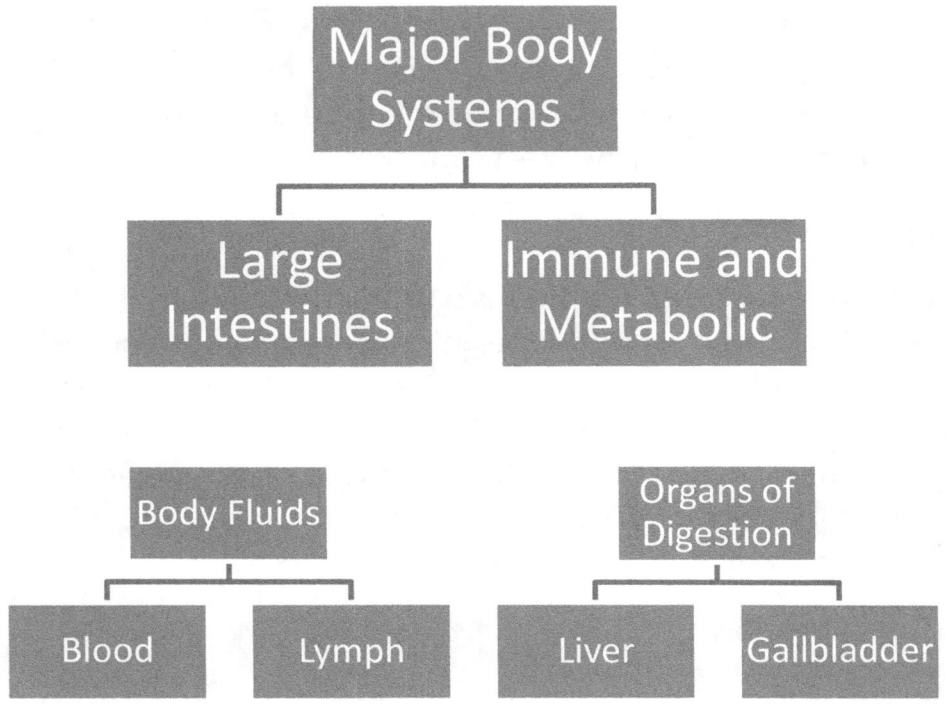

Beauty is only skin deep. Cleansing is the real Key to beauty enhancing health in the body systems achieves beauty from the inside out. Detoxify your body, cleanse and protect it from Dis -Ease.

CLEANSING AND DETOXIFICATION, PART 1

Please answer the following questions.

Why make a commitment to cleanse and detoxify?

_____
_____
_____
_____
_____
_____
_____

How can you benefit from this natural healing plan?

_____
_____
_____
_____
_____
_____
_____

What outcome do you expect?

_____
_____
_____
_____
_____
_____

YOU MAY INSERT A RECENT PICTURE OF YOURSELF:

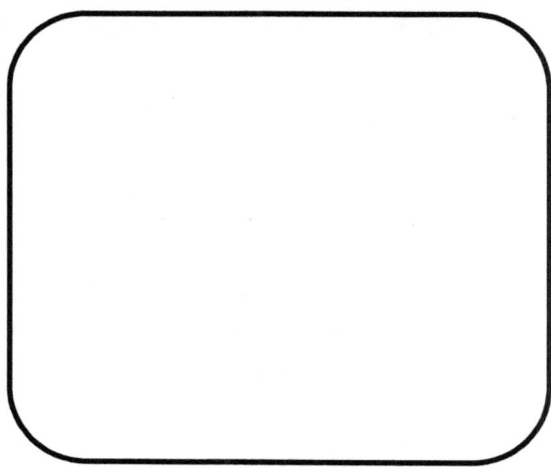

SKETCH WHAT YOU WANT TO LOOK LIKE IN THE FUTURE:

What do you understand about the phrase, "beauty is skin deep"?

_____
_____
_____
_____
_____
_____

WHAT IS YOUR COMMITMENT to STICK-TO-IT?

(List 5 steps that will help)

1.

2.

3.

4.

5.

Sign and date to confirm your commitment:

X
_____

Act as if "THIS IS THE FIRST DAY OF the REST OF YOUR LIFE."

You have arrived at a point of your life where cleansing is most urgent to restore, and renew your health.

CLEANSING AND DETOXIFICATION, PART 2

Detoxification is a safe and a most natural way to restore improve and rejuvenate your health. However, it is often overlooked by many, including the health professionals. We must acknowledge that a sick body is a toxic body. Toxic acids are normal end-products of cell catabolism. We assimilate toxic material from the air we breathe, the water we drink, the foods we eat and other environmental sources.

There is no problem when toxic material can be eliminated from the body; however, when such is accumulated faster than when it can be moved out then there is an increasing problem. Similarly, when some organs of elimination are blocked the body malfunctions and disease develops.

Our bodies become overwhelmed by toxic accumulations as a consequence of fatigue, poor circulation and improper diet. A sluggish and clogged up body system is burdened by toxins and does not have the capacity to get rid of toxic waste material. The more toxic waste remaining in the body, the less oxygen goes to the cells. We cannot throw off toxins without enough oxygen in the body tissues. As a result, sick people are always tired and out of sorts.

MAJOR CAUSES BEHIND ALL FAILING HEALTH

- Lack of the correct combination of nutrients

- Lack of oxygen at a cellular level including the ability of the cells to utilize oxygen

- Accumulation of toxins, poisons and waste because of an inability of the body to detoxify.

- Increase stressors causing lowered vitality e.g. Injury, losses, relationship problems, emotional upsets.

- Poor dietary food intake and nutritional status; which many times acquired from birth.

LAUGHTER IS ESSENTIAL

A Laugh a Day: According to new medicals research, the old adage, "An apple a day keeps the doctor away," may be changed to "laugh (or two) a day keeps the doctor away."

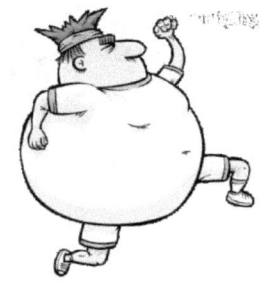

"My doctor took one look at my gut and refused to believe that I work out. So I listed the exercises I do every day: jump to conclusions, climb the walls, drag my heels, push my luck, make mountains out of molehills, bend over backward, run around in circles, put my foot in my mouth, go over the edge, and beat around the bush."

– From *Reader's Digest*

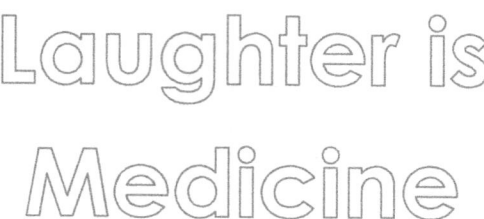

SELF-ASSESSMENT TOOL

Self-Assessment Tools: Assess Your Toxic Load: Please answer the following questions as truthfully as you can. Score one point for every YES and a 0 for NO. Unless you score a 5 points or less, you should break yourself in gently.

There is no right or wrong score here, but you should keep score so that you can measure your progress after completing the detoxification procedure. Your healing journey starts today, right here!

Write in **yes** or **no** next to each question.

1. Do you feel tired when you wake up in the morning, even though you've enough sleep?

2. Do you drink more than 3 cups of coffee, tea or caffeinated fizzy drinks such as cola or coke every day?

3. Do you suffer skin rashes, spots, eczema or cracked areas around the mouth?

4. Do you have bloating after meals?

5. Do you have alcoholic drink most days?

6. Do you smoke or live with smokers?

7. Do you use pesticides in your living or work environment?

8. Do you rarely eat fresh fruits and vegetables?

9. Do you eat red meat, chicken or fish more than twice a week?

10. Do you eat fried foods and/or junk foods?

11. Do you suffer constant colds/flu, allergies or hay fever?

12. Do you feel irritable easily or have angry outbursts for little or/no reason?

13. Do you have mood swings?

14. Do you crave certain foods, such as candy, coffee, or baked goods?

15. Do you skip meals, especially breakfast or because of stomach upset?

16. Do you gain weight easily?

17. Do you find it difficult to concentrate?

18. Do you regularly have 2 or 3 bowel movements every day?

19. Do you take laxatives often for constipation or medicines for diarrhea?

20. Do your joints or muscles sometimes ache?

21. Do you feel tired and lethargic most of the time?

22. Do you observe a white coating over your tongue?

23. Do you have bad breath or a foul body odor?

24. Do you suffer from fungal infections, such as thrush, athletes' foot, ringworm or jock itch?

25. Do you have white spots on your face or skin areas?

SCORE

YES = 1   **NO = 0**   **YOUR RESULT =**

_____

A, B, Cs OF LOSING WEIGHT AND KEEPING IT OFF

Activate your body clock

Balance body cells

Cleanse and detoxify

Direct and release ailments

Exercise consciously, stretching and relaxing the large muscles

Losing weight and keeping it off involves these important factors, proper nutritional health, managing emotions and a total change in lifestyle. This will bring you the best results to reach your identified goals. Remember it took you a long time to get to where you are now and it will take a while to achieve that desired goal. Be patient with yourself. There is no quick fix, however with conscientious and diligent effort you will get the best body you want and will keep the weight off.

Here are steps to get there!

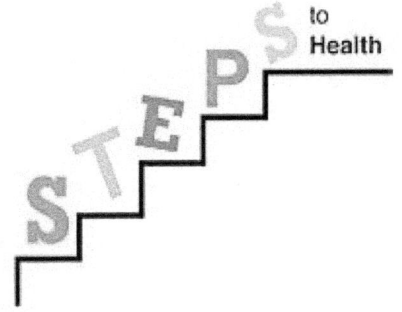

STEPS to Health

Cleanse the body.

Relax the mind.

Renew the spirit.

CHECK THIS OUT FOR YOURSELF TO SEE IF YOU NEED TO CLEANSE AND DETOXIFY:

Do you experience any of the following?

- feeling stuffed up?
- constipated, irregular bowel movements?
- dull headaches?
- sinuses congested?
- gas and bloated?
- heartburn or acid reflux?
- bad breath and/or poor body odor?
- tongue coated white?
- overweight and tired?
- low energy and depressed?
- suffering many ailments?
- muscle and joint aches and pains?

If you answered yes to any of these questions, then you may consider an appointment for the Cleansing and Detoxification Regimen.

Restore and rejuvenate the whole person and see how fantastic you feel. You may like the new you even better.

HEALTHFUL BENEFITS OF COLON HYDROTHERAPY

When the colon is cleansed adequately, Vitamin A can be more effectively absorbed through the intestinal tract. Colon irrigation may help greatly in enhancing the body's ability to absorb many vitamins, minerals, essential fatty acids; especially the macro and micro-nutrients that the body needs to sustain good health.

Also, colonics may perform a very important function in helping to expel toxins from the body. Many health authorities believe that constipation is the number one affliction of our civilized world and it under- lies nearly every ailment known to mankind.

Constipation contributes toward the lowering of the body's resistance predisposing it to many acute illnesses and the beginnings of many degenerative and chronic diseases. A malfunctioning colon is unable to perform efficiently and regularly.

Therefore, hard fecal matter lodges and creates both intestinal constipation and toxic overload in many organs. This in turn increases the workload of the eliminatory organs, e.g. kidneys, skin, lymph, liver and the lungs.

Many health conscious people ask how to eliminate mucous formed in the body systems. The best way to begin is by eliminating mucoid forming foods and to move gradually to a toxic less diet. Freely use vegetables, fruits, sprouts, honey, maple syrup, millet, once a day and supplements such as kelp and zinc.

Millet grain is gluten free and is less mucoid forming than wheat, rice, oats, rye or barley. Millet controls the aggressive cleansing activity of fruits, vegetables and honey. Example of a toxicless diet using Millet is best prepared in the following way: See Recipes.

PREPARATION

Goats' milk products are far better substitutes than dairy products from cows' milk.

CONSTIPATION:

Difficult defecation or passage of stools, Infrequent passage of hard, dry, fecal material. The bowel is sluggish, sometimes the person experiences bloating, gas, fecal odor and discomfort while trying to have a bowel movement.

COLONIC IRRIGATION

This is a hygienic procedure that cleanses the lower bowel or colon, by infusing water into the rectum.

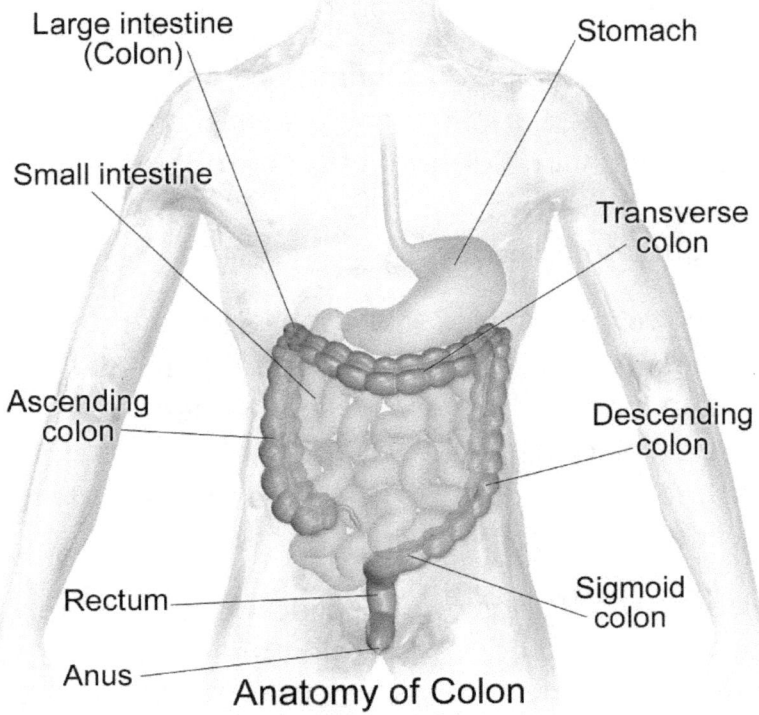

Anatomy of Colon

Colon irrigation is different from an enema, in that an enema only clears feces from the Rectum, wherein a Colonic Irrigation clears and cleanses the Large Intestines of fecal waste material. Colonic Irrigation has been practiced in Europe and used to promote good health for centuries in many parts of the world.

What are the benefits of colon irrigation?

- Promotes self-healing, detoxification and weight problems.
- Stimulates bowel function
- Helps to restore and maintain better health.

Who should have colon irrigations?

- Anyone experiencing common ailments, such as constipation, sluggish digestion, sinus problems
- Preparation for diagnostic studies such as Barium Enema, Colonoscopy.
- Weight control problems

How to prepare: A 5-day preparation is recommended to prepare for a colonic irrigation. Eat 80% raw foods that include fresh fruits and vegetables e.g. watermelon, cantaloupe, spinach, carrots, avocado, broccoli, limes and grapefruit, to name a few. Doing this helps the body to change from acidic to alkalinity.

Drink at least 8 to 10 glasses of purified water daily and fresh squeezed juices. Contact your colon Therapist for complete guidelines (New Body Protocol). COLONIC IRRIGATION is intended as a preventive and cleansing measure to good health... It is not a medical procedure nor is it intended in anyway to be used as a substitute for medical care.

COLON IRRIGATION WITH EUNICE M. CLARKE

Cleanse the colon and see how fantastic you feel!

- Feeling all stuffed up?
- Sinuses congested?
- Constipated, depressed?
- Dull headaches?
- Bad breath?
- Gas and bloated?
- Weight gain?
- Aches and pains?

What's Included?

- Digestive system assessment
- Colon cleanse/care
- Pre-diagnostic screening
- Nutritional assessment
- Acid/alkaline balance
- Food Combining
- Mental Health Counseling

If you have medical problems discuss this with your therapist beforehand or see your medical doctor who will establish a plan of care.

Schedule your colon irrigation or Healing Journey in Bullet Tree Falls, Belize. Accommodations available.

Email: essai963c@yahoo.com
Eunice Clarke, M.A., BSN
Colon Hydrotherapist, Certified

Try Colon Irrigation to improve your health.

We use the closed system Toxygen Equipment.

If you have medical problems discuss this with your therapist beforehand or see your medical doctor who will establish a plan of care.

PREPARATION FOR THE COLON IRRIGATION PROCEDURE

Prepare and Drink laxative tea for 3 nights before having the Procedure. Prepare: ¼ oz Senna Leaves and 1 handful Cerosi leaves and stem. Boil in 10 ounces of water for 5 minutes, turn off the fire, cover and allow tea to steep. Drink when cool.

THE NIGHT BEFORE YOUR COLON IRRIGATION: Nothing to eat after 6pm.

May drink Tea and Water if desired.

Do not have breakfast prior to the Colon Irrigation.

Your plan may be: A one-time Lower Bowel Cleanse and Colon irrigation session or the 7 to 10 day Healing Journey. Each plan Requires a different protocol and preparation.

Your individualized plan will be discussed with you in detail by your Holistic Practitioner.

YOUR TONGUE: A MAGIC MIRROR

"The surface of the tongue indicates the appearance of the inside of the body... Nature shows and plainly reveals and shows everything exact and perfect than all the sciences of diagnostics put together." By: Prof. Arnold Ehret; 1953

The tongue should be pink and without a coating and the breath without bad odor.

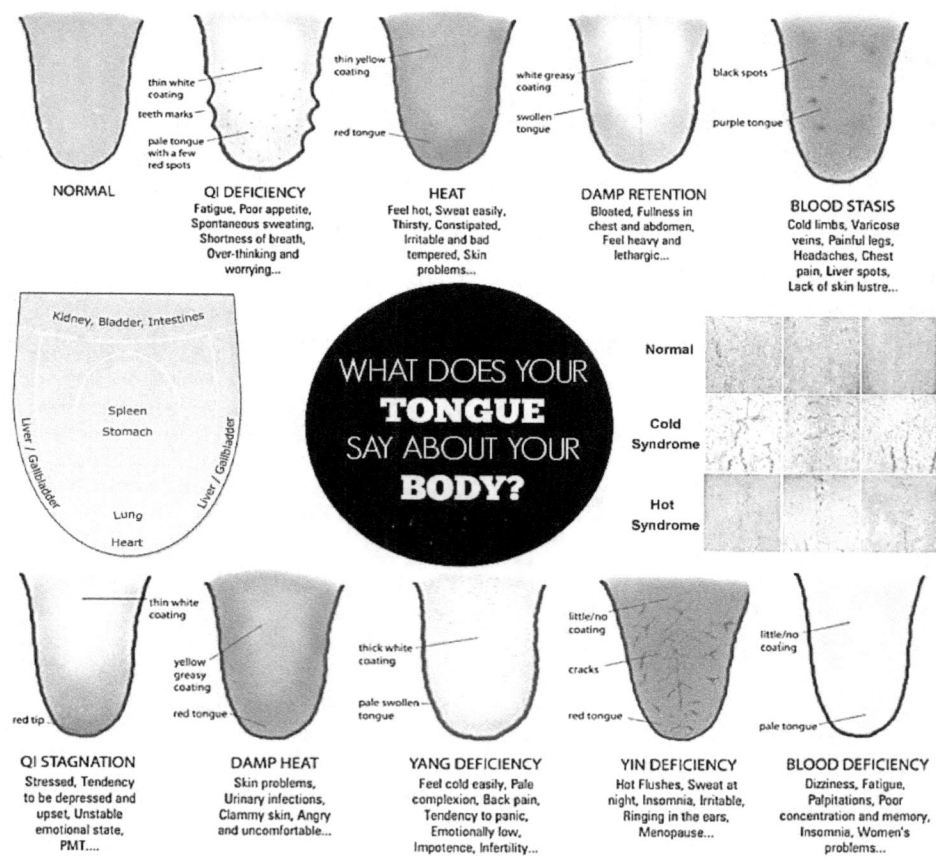

ABCD's OF LIFESTYLE CHANGE

Do you know that many symptoms could be the cause to toxic buildup in the body? Ailments and complaints such as: Menstrual/female problems; skin problems; allergies/allergic reactions; constipation; gas/bloating, backache, frequent colds/flu; sinus and lung congestion; bad breath, coated tongue; forgetfulness/poor memory; anxiety/ worry/tension; headaches; low energy/fatigue; overweight; overeating etc. lack of sexual response; and many more. These are some of the reasons why thousands of people each year choose to detox and change their eating habits, together with Colon Irrigation to assist in the cleansing process!

YOUR HEALTH IS YOUR WEALTH!

How much value does it have?

How much value do you place on having good health?

Cleansing and detoxing, keep the bowels moving and keeps the system clean. Many research facts show that at least 96% of disease begin in the colon. Cleaning out the colon begins the cleansing process and makes detoxifying the cells effective.

TIPS: WHERE TO BEGIN... Consider the Natural A-B-C and D of Natural Healing for your body. **A**ctivate your body, **B**uild the body cells, **C**leanse your body cells 2 to 4 times a year, **D**irect help for an ailment.

Losing weight and keeping it off involves five important factors.

1. Proper nutrition. 2. Conscientious exercise. 3. Managing emotions 4. Internal cleansing 5. Change of lifestyle.

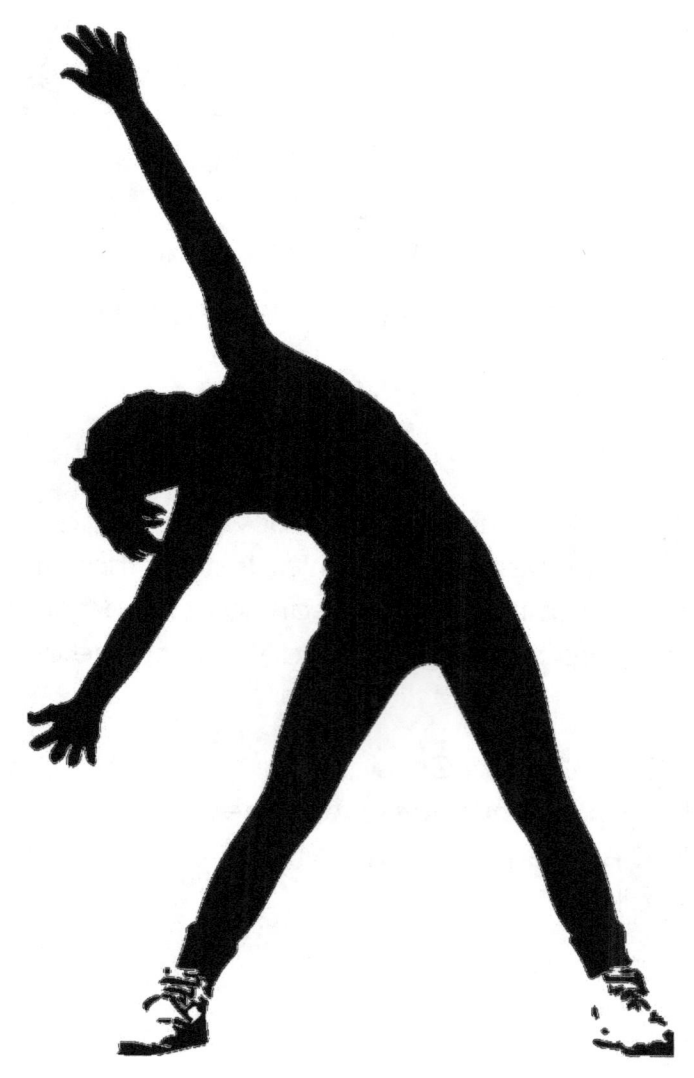

EEEEEEEEEs OF LIFESTYLE CHANGE 4 EXAMINE GET RID OF UNWANTED STUFF.

1.) EAT

YOU ARE WHAT YOU EAT. Good and healthy foods are building blocks for the physical body. If we are to enjoy good health foods must be selected to provide the nutrients the body requires rather than to indulge the appetite and use only what "taste good."

Anytime we overeat, or eat fried or processed foods together with being exposed to continued stressors and pollutants from the environment, the liver becomes extremely overtaxed and has difficulty processing toxins and fats efficiently.

Consider an intake of healthy healing foods e.g. all dark green foods are alive and revive the body cells. A daily food intake should consist of fruits, vegetable, grains, seeds with the vitamins and minerals needed to metabolize them and help to revive and rejuvenate the body.

Water provides bulk in the diet helping the body to cleanse, promotes regularity for the intestinal tract and energizes the whole system. The use of water: Your body is approximately 60% of water. The cells of the body contain and must be bathed daily in various fluids which are mostly water.

Body fluids carry nutrients into the cells and remove waste material, carrying it away for elimination. Water is necessary for the production of digestive juices and the healthy action of the stomach and intestines. Drink lots of water to flush the body cells. Take at least 6 to 8 glasses of purified water daily.

2.) ELIMINATE

WHAT GOES IN MUST COME OUT. Anytime you take in two and more solid meals daily, you should have at least 2 formed bowel movements every day. Daily elimination of the bowel helps the body to flush out toxic waste products.

Stools should be firm and moist, not hard and dry. Hard, dry stools indicate constipation. Stools should float in the toilet bowl and should not contain bright red blood (hemorrhoids), black tarry (intestinal bleeding). Elimination should not be putrid or high smelling and should not be painful at any time.

3.) EXERCISE

MOVE IT OR LOSE IT. Exercise is mainly to build, trim, tone, strengthen and controlling body weight. Inactivity or lack of exercise causes pain and stiffness, rust and corrosion in the joints, decreased energy and worst of all, sluggishness of the colon…You become a Couch Potato.

So commit to keeping the muscles energized and supple through exercise. 20 TO 25 MINUTES OF SUSTAINED MOVEMENT 3 TO 4 TIMES WEEKLY will help to keep you or the right track. Move the muscles and help the body to get rid of toxins/poisons, through the skin by perspiration, from the lungs by deep breathing, from the kidneys by urination, and from the colon by regular bowel movements.

Activities recommended include walking, running, swimming, bicycling, yoga to name a few.

4.) EXAMINE

GET RID OF UNWANTED STUFF. This unwanted STUFF is anything that is no longer useful in your life or for your good, be it persons, places, conditions or things. Example: Clothing, shoes, jewelry, that you have not used for one year or more. Find and associate with new friends. Get rid of those who "sap your energy."

Clean house. Learn and practice something new, daily. Reconnect with someone who you have been out of contact. Forgive those who have hurt you or you have hurt them, for whatever the reason may be.

5.) ENRICH

AS WE THINK SO WE BECOME. Seek knowledge and information. Must watch how we use our EYES... they are the DOORWAY TO THE SOUL. Guard the hearing, Gossip------NO, NO!!!!! Watch our words, they create thought forms and return to SENDER. Practice: HEAR NO EVIL, SEE NO EVIL, SPEAK NO EVIL. Everything we say and do records in the body.

6.) EASE STRESS

KEEP THINGS SIMPLE!

Establish a good sleep pattern; prepare the body for sleep, e.g.: wear comfortable clothing, turn off noise including television. Plan time to relax and release by taking deep breaths, inhale and exhale for a 20-minute cycle. By exhaling, you release fear from the body, because pent up fear causes pain in the muscles. So practice concentrated breathing and releasing for 10 to 15 minutes before sleep every night. YOU'LL SLEEP LIKE A BABY.

7.) ELIMINATE

THINK OFTEN ON YOUR HIGHEST GOOD.

Contemplate your creator, nature, birds, animals, bees, the little ant. There is much to learn from them.

Adopt a child, a pet, or start a hobby (something that you wanted to create that will be of help to others). Meditate, go within, find and discover your God-self, your strength, the source of your being.

Find out something new about you, EVERY DAY...do you like it? If not change it and find the new you. Be grateful for life daily. Smile more often. LIFE IS GOOD. Keep a journal write in it at the end of each day.

8.) ENJOY

RADIATE LOVE AND PEACE: Eliminate gossips, envy, jealousy, hatred. These are toxic poisons too. Find your true inner child and love him/her Stand in front of a mirror and give yourself HUGS daily Smile, sing, and dance (not only from the music outside, you will also find sweetness coming from within). Allow others to assist you on your Healing Journey of body, mind, and spirit. Give back to life more. Share what you have with others and life will give back to you.

The laws of Giving and Receiving are like the ebb and flow of the ocean cycle. These are the Essssssssssssssssssss OF A LIFESTYLE CHANGE. Ease the mind, Renew the SPIRIT, Nourish the BODY. CLEANSING AND DETOXIFICATION must take place in the mind, the spirit when complete, change will manifest in the body.

THE RAINBOW FOOD OF LIFE based on the colors of the rainbow.

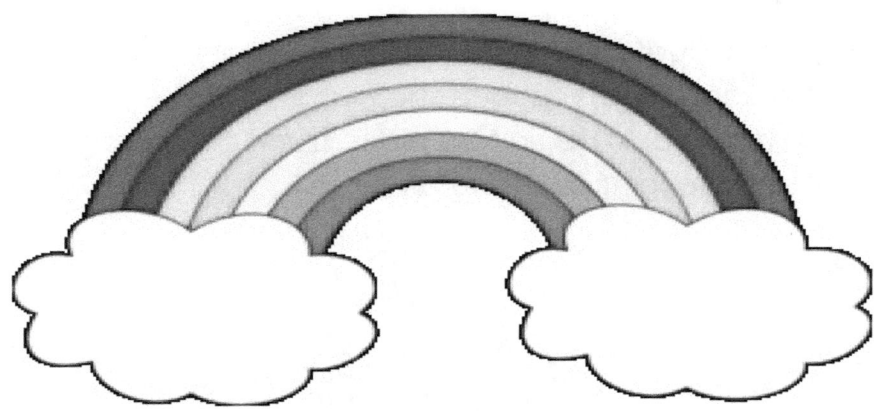

White: All white foods of roots and vegetables, Milk- only for the infant.

GOAT MILK: an ideal food, the closest to human milk. It is a food that nourishes the brain, high in chlorine and effective in kidney disturbance because of its germicidal properties. (Bernard Jensen, 1978) Milk, the food of the Mother.

Violet, Indigo, Blue: Berries and fruits, growing high off the ground, reaching for the spirit.

Green: Vegetables and weeds of the sea, healing me.

Yellow: Grains, eggs, cheese, butter, and oils golden gifts of substance range: Carrots, pumpkin, and squash, citrus and melons, rich in the power of life

Red: and if there is a need to ground the self, to stabilize and warm the fragile body, use hot and spicy cook the foods in the blessing of fire.

Cooking and eating can be a ritual of love for Mother Earth, Spirit, and Self. The more you appreciate and bless your food, the more it will bless you. If you eat from the rainbow of life-giving substances, you will seldom have to deal with illness.

If you are habituated to cigarettes, coffee, alcohol, medical or nonmedical drugs, or sugar and highly processed, chemicalized foods, begin to replace them one by one with a food from the rainbow of life.

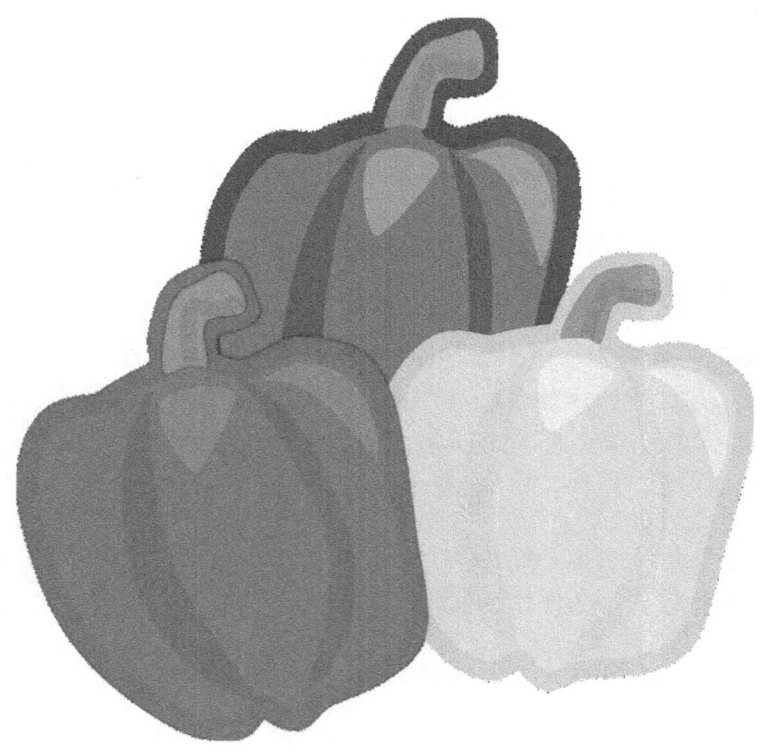

The Food Rainbow of Life

Every time you indulge in an old habit or substance, do it in a prayerful way, such as:

"Creator within me, I offer you this habit that it might lead me to transformation. I bless this substance for what it has given me and ask to be easily and quickly show that which must now replace it."

On the physical level, eat the freshest, most wholesome foods that are closest to their natural states. Eat foods that are available and in season. Whenever possible, eat the foods that are in season and grown close to home. This keeps your vibration in tune with your environment.

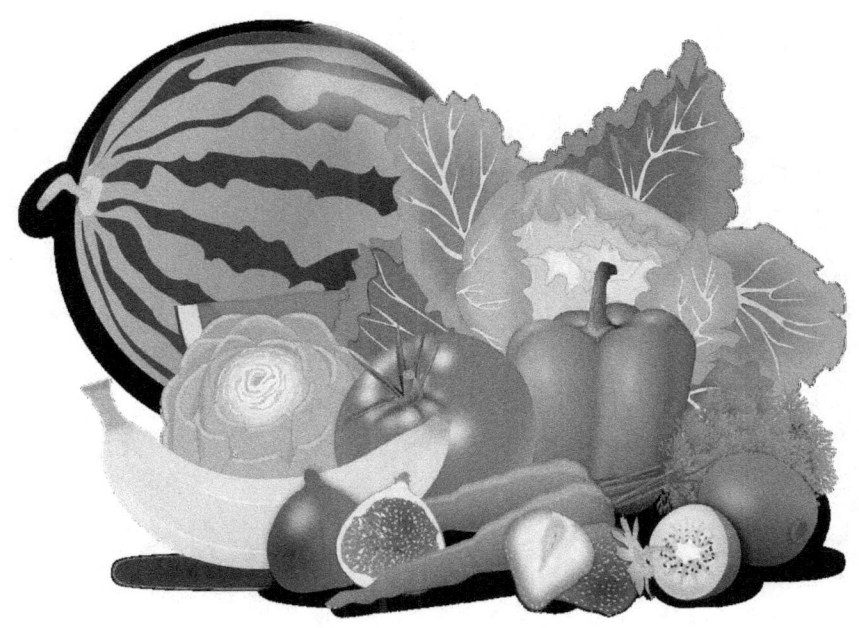

Clip the following verse and put it on your refrigerator to remind you of these lessons.

> Sun is the first food,
> Fresh air and water second,
> Rest, exercise, and laughter,
> Nourish you, third,
> Fourth, the seed of Earth brings life,
> Fifth, the herb, vegetable, and fruit give health,
> Sixth, if these be lacking,
> The animals will provide,
> Cast aside as little as you can
> From these, the gifts that nourish,
> This, is thanksgiving for their being;
>
> Be positive and kind in preparation
> Friendly and serene in consuming,
> Joyful and active in digestion,
> And health will be your inner light,
> Eat from nature, if you can,
> The herbs and wild foods provided,
> Garden by organic means or purchase,
> The least affected, neglected, processed, and imperfected,
> Locally grown helps you be tuned to home,
> Above all, envision
> Radiant vitality to be your own.

NATURE HAS A REMEDY

Orange represents grains. The USDA recommends eating 5-8 ounces of grain per day depending on your age and gender. Of that amount, at least 3 ounces should be whole grain breads, crackers, pasta, cereals or rice.

Green represents vegetables. The USDA's dietary guidelines recommend 2½ cups of vegetables per day for people eating 2,000 calories a day, with higher or lower amounts depending on the calories level. People are urged to select from all five vegetable subgroups (dark green, orange, legumes, starchy vegetables, and other vegetables) several times a week.

Red represents fruits. The latest dietary guidelines call for people to eat two cups of fruit a day.

Yellow represents oil. The USDA recommends getting most of your fat source from fish, nuts and vegetable oils, and limiting solid fats like butter, stick margarine, lard and shortening.

Blue represents milk. The latest USDA dietary guidelines encourage consuming three cups per day of fat free or low-fat milk or equivalent milk products every day.

Purple represents beams and meats. The USDA says people should choose lean meats and poultry, varying protein choices with more fish, beans, peas, nuts and seeds.

GOAT MILK: an ideal food, the closest to human milk. It is a brain food, high in chlorine and is effective in kidney disturbances because of its germicide effects. (Bernard Jensen, 1978)

COMMITMENT TO YOUR GOOD HEALTH

When a vehicle's engine is full of carbon, it is hard to start and has no pep. The internal systems are clogged up. The most logical thing to do is to have the carbon cleaned out. Then there is plenty of power to move around. That is like cleansing and detoxifying your body systems. Similarly, the body can be compared to such a vehicle. When the body systems, including organs, cells and tissues become carbonized and clogged up with acid-sugar-mucus-pus. Etc.

The real problem is, TOXIC OVERLOAD!

- Your appetite is poor
- You do not sleep well
- Your complexion is sallow and bad
- Your eyes are dull
- You have many aches and pains
- You feel sad and often overeat
- You need a strong drink every night to relax and one to start the day
- You are nervous, irritable, anxious, you lack "gusto" and interest in life
- Nothing makes you feel happy and everything seems wrong
- Your skin with spots, blotches and discoloration

To sum it all up, LIFE IS JUST NOT WHAT IT USED TO BE, for you. You are really ill.

The most sensible and logical thing to do, is to CLEAN OUT and CLEAR UP, not only the bowels but the systemic cells. Go to the root cause of the problem. Get all the accumulated toxic material out. Detoxify to improve your health.

The Goal: To recharge and keep all body systems working in harmony.

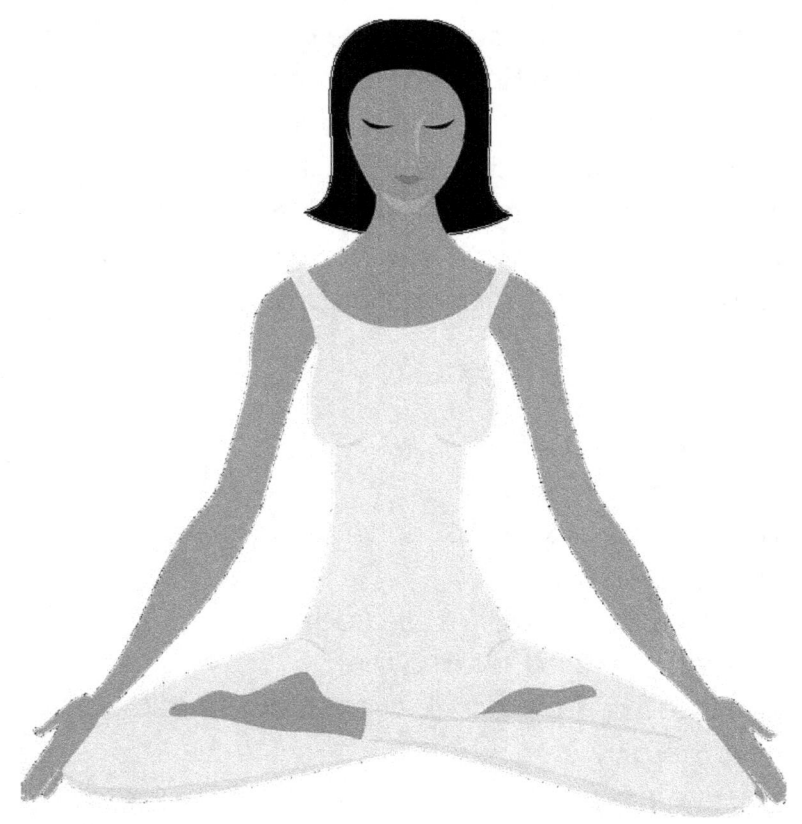

Daily water consumption helps to flush out toxins from the body. It is better to drink an extra glass of water to avoid eating when you are not hungry. Do this before preparing a snack or a meal. If within half an hour the hunger does not subside, then it is okay to eat a meal.

Drink 8 to 10 glasses of pure water daily.

Drink fresh natural juices whenever possible.

Eat at least 80% fresh fruits and raw vegetables.

Cold drinks should be taken at rooms temperature and not ice cold.

For sweeteners, use brown sugar, maple syrup or molasses. No white sugar.

Carrot juice is nutritious and wonderful for the body but it is high in sugar content. Make carrot juice: add an apple, a slice of white ginger, lime juice with a small piece of sweet potato. This makes a satisfying and pleas- ant beverage snack. Even children love this drink. If you need to restrict sugar intake, you should dilute carrot juice with other vegetable juices or water. Use citrus fruit by themselves. Do not mix with other fruits and vegetables.

ACID-ALKALINE BALANCE

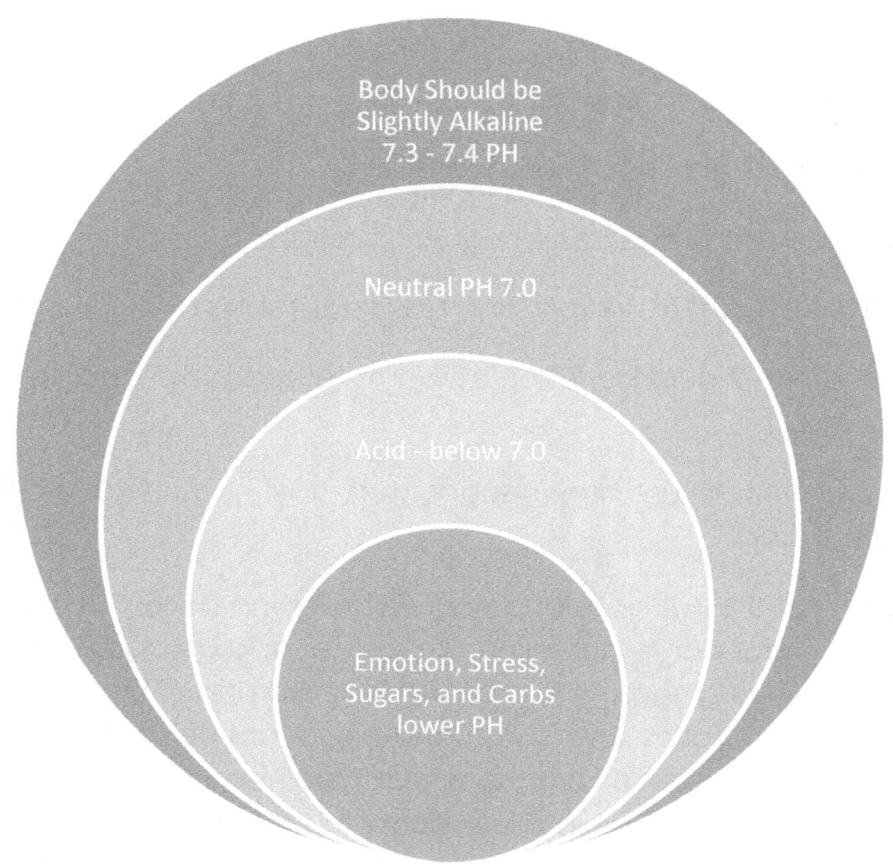

Acid forming diet acidic, with a PH that is below 7.0 Emotion and stress Lower PH level also Sugars and all Carbohydrates cause Toxic overload lower blood PH level.

Any process that deprives cells of O2 (oxygen) and nutrients creates an acid environment. The body will try to compensate in attempt to re-balance. By using alkaline minerals e.g. Potassium will help to balance the body's PH. If the diet does not have enough minerals, then a buildup of acids will take place in the cells.

Acid imbalance:

- poor absorption of minerals and nutrients
- decrease energy produced in cells.
- decreased ability of cell repair. (repairing damaged cells)
- ability to detox heavy metals
- formation of tumor cells, fatigue, and illness.

A blood PH of solid acid can lead to coma and death.

Reason: Our diet is mainly more acid than alkaline e.g. animal products = meat, eggs, dairy, white flour, coffee, carbonated beverages and processed foods create acidic levels in the blood.

High alkaline foods such as fresh fruits and dark green leafy vegetables offer the best protection from acidity.

Drugs are acid forming and metallic same as artificial sweeteners. Best way to correct acidity is to Cleanse and Detoxify through a dietary regimen and a total change in lifestyle.

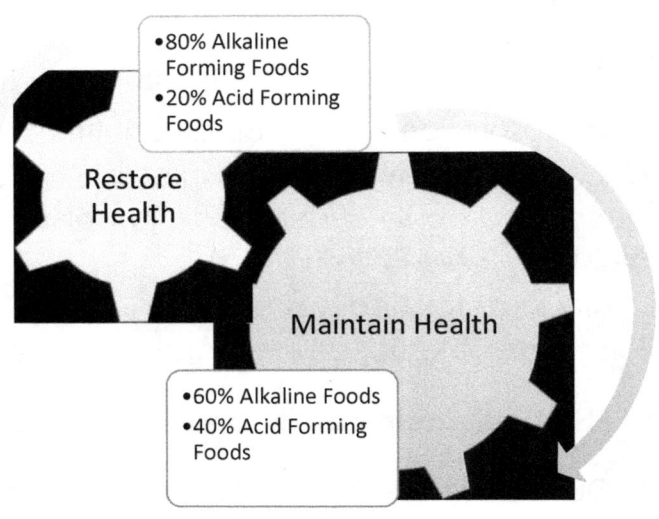

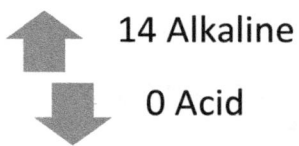 14 Alkaline

0 Acid

7.0 PH Balance

Examples of levels:

1. Battery
2. Lemon Juice
3. Vinegar
4-5. Weaker Strengths
6. Milk
7-8. Baking Soda

9. Sea Water
10. Milk of Magnesia
11-12. Ammonia
13. Lye

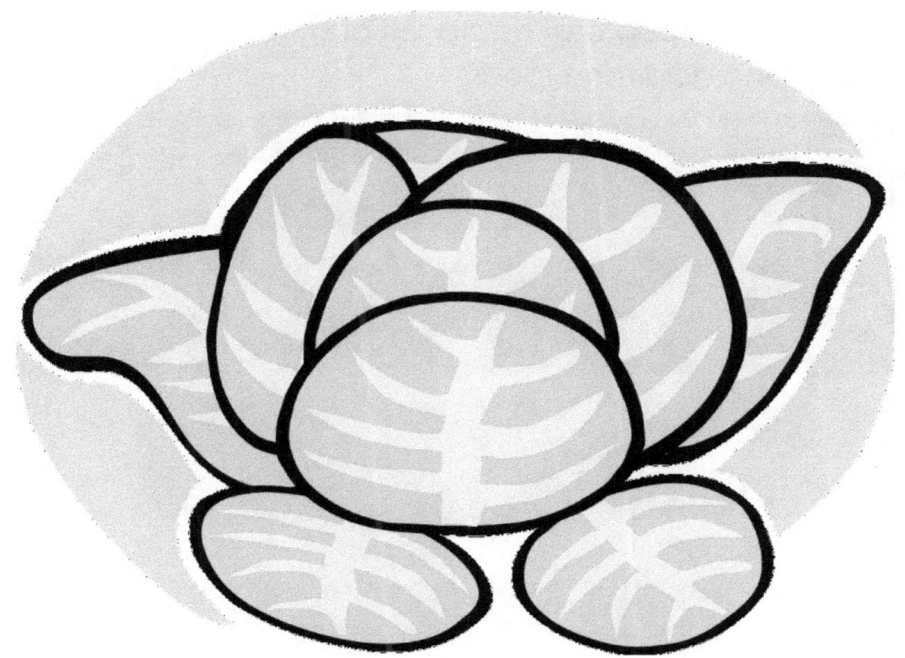

Generally, alkaline forming foods include; most fruits, green leafy vegetables, peas, beans, lentils, spices, herbs and seasoning, and seeds and nuts.

Generally, acid forming foods include; meat, fish poultry, eggs, grains, and legumes.

Shift your pH toward Alkaline.

An acidic body is a sickness magnet. What you eat and drink will impact where your body's pH level falls; balance or imbalance.

This chart is intended only as a point of general reference to alkalizing and acidifying foods:

ALKALINE VEGETABLES	Beet Greens	Beets	Broccoli
Cabbage	Carrot	Cauliflower	Celery
	Chard Greens	Chlorella	Collard Greens

ACIDIFYING VEGETABLES	Corn	Lentils	Olives	Winter Squash

ACIDIFYING FRUITS	Blueberries	Canned or Glazed fruits
Cranberries	Currants	Prunes

ACIDIFYING GRAINS	Amaranth	Barley	Bran	Oat Bran
Wheat Bread	Corn	Cornstarch	Soda Crackers	Wheat Flour
		White Flour		

56

MAKE A CONSCIOUS COMMITMENT TO FOLLOW THIS REGIMEN FOR THE NEXT 90 DAYS.

This regimen is to help you to cleanse the body of mucus, toxins and expel fecal material, schedule quality quiet time daily for yourself, meditation, reading, music

Keep a Journal on your progress, loving yourself for each step achieved.

THIS IS THE ONLY BODY YOU WERE GIVEN, A TEMPLE, WITH ALL THE EQUIPMENT TO LIVE OVER 100 YEARS. SO TREASURE IT!

YOU WILL BE ON LIVE HEALING FOODS TO BRING THE BODY ORGANS BACK INTO BALANCE, FROM ACID TO ALKALINE:

6 AM: CITRUS POWER (ORANGE JUICE)
8 AM: BREAKFAST IN A CUP (OATMEAL AND FRUIT)
10 AM: GREEN POWER MIX (LEAFY GREENS)
12 NOON: CRUNCHY LUNCH (ALKALINE VEGETABLES)
 PM: GREEN POWER MIX (ALKALINE GREENS)
4 PM: CITRUS POWER (ORANGE JUICE)
6 PM: GREEN POWER MIX (ALKALINE GREENS)
8 PM: TEA TIME (HERBAL TEA)
9 PM: LUBE LOB (DRINKING OLIVE OIL WITH LIME JUICE AND WATER BEFORE BED)

BEDTIME: RELAX, RENEW, REJOICE:

AT HOME: IT IS RECOMMENDED TO USE FRESH FRUITS AND VEGETABLES HAVE EVERY THING READY AVAILABLE AND IN THE HOUSE TO PREPARE SHAKES, SALADS AND CITRUS DRINKS ETC.

BODY CLEANSING: FROM ACIDIC TO ALKALINE:

1 GRAPEFRUIT, 1 LEMON/LIME, 1 ORANGE, IF ANY FRUIT IS UNAVAILABLE, THEN DOUBLE UP ON ONE OF THE OTHERS.

MOLASSES 1 TABLESPOON, NONI 1 TABLESPOON, HONEY IF DESIRED. ADD WARM WATER FOR A TOTAL PINT OF MIXTURE. SIP SLOWLY ALL IN 5 MINUTES. BREAKFAST IN A CUP

CRUNCHY LUNCH: Salad greens Cucumber, cabbage, tomatoes, beets, fresh green beans, black beans Vinegar, mustard, Bragg amino, olive oil, ¼ tsp cayenne powder Mix together in a bowl. Allow to sit for at least 1 hour before eating

Succotash bean salad: ½ cup soaked black beans, 1 cup is pollun beans, CILANTRO ½ tsp white ginger 1 tablespoonful BRAGG AMINO, 1 tablespoonful VIRGIN OLIVE OIL 1 CUPFUL COOKED BROWN RICE GREEN POWER MIX: Blend: Spinach, ½ tsp Spurillina,, Carrot, 3 celery stalks, ½ ripe plantain, 1 small sweet potato 8 ounces water, 1 tsp Apple Cider Vinegar, Honey if desired. 24 25

SOME FIRST AID REMEDIES THAT PROMOTE GOOD HEALTH

Bless everything that enters your mouth, even a glass of water.

Every organ is represented on the tongue.

Inspect the tongue and clean it every morning.

No gossip, slander or back talking. This creates severe life penalties for the sender.

Send loving thoughts to all the parts of the body, thank it for functioning faithfully. Example: eyes for sight, ears for hearing mouth tongue teeth etc. Thank the heart for being on-time with regular beats. Lungs, breaths - inhaling and exhaling. The liver, breaking down and storing. Intestines - absorbing nutrients. Colon, skin, and kidneys - being the most efficient garbage disposable system; collecting and eliminating waste and toxins Feet and hands - doing for and transporting you with no questions asked.

Malfunction, pain, discomfort etc. send love and kindness to the part.

Having headaches, use trigger points between the eyes or points between the thumb and forefinger.

Give a loving belly rub to the colon every morning before hopping out of bed.

Take a deep breath and greet the sun to acknowledge its presence.

Pamper self and reverse your age.

Perform foot care; massage feet pay attention to the heels and toes. Use warm water with Epsom Salt and a little vinegar added.

Do facial massage 5 to 10 minutes daily after brushing your (mouth of pearls) teeth.

Smile a lot Don't frown-you will have no worry lines and you will erase any crow's feet.

Steam the face, move the muscles up toward hairline.

Use apple cider vinegar in bath water.

Use baking soda to brush your teeth of pearls, and eliminate mouth odors.

Baking soda also works eliminates underarm and body odors.

Do not allow anyone who is angry or blowing of cigarette smoke, do your hair care etc.

Perform breast self-examination monthly; this applies to both male and female.

Seek professional advice for any abnormalities found. Males should perform monthly scrotal examinations also.

Pay attention to your prostate and your breathing.

Take time to uplift your spirit within the vehicle that houses it.

Feed your spirit with all that is Good, Tender, and Loving.

Nurture and uplift your mind. Think no evil, see no evil, hear no evil, speak no evil.

These are guard and guides at your life's gate.

Feed the spirit, and Be Always Grateful. look around, there is someone worse off than you.

Nourish the physical body with the best nutrition foods. You become what you eat!

Keep your life fulfilled. Only you are responsible for your happiness.

LIVE, LAUGH LOVE AND PLAY. Lighten up! That's all that matters......

BENEFITS OF CITRUS JUICE: LEMON/ LIME CITRUS

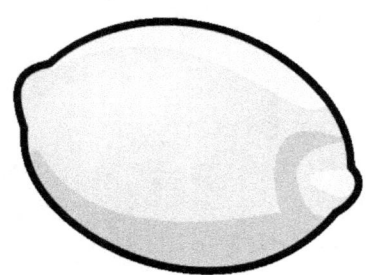

According to a 2010 study conducted by Mario Ferruzzi, assistant professor of food science at Purdue University, lemon juice added to green tea can increase the amount of antioxidants available to your body.

Catechins, antioxidants found in green tea" tend to lose their ability to be absorbed once they reach the intestines. The addition of citrus juice, such as lemon or lime juice left 80 percent of the tea's Catechins available for absorption in a simulated model.

Citrus juices contain large amounts of vitamin C, a water soluble nutrient necessary for the formation of collagen, bones, muscles, blood and cartilage. Vitamin C also helps your body absorb iron. Because bile from the gallbladder is released when you eat food containing fat, drinking water with lemon juice and olive oil may help you expel gallstones.

Article by: Jason Marcus, June 14, 2011: Institute of Nutrition Education and Research.

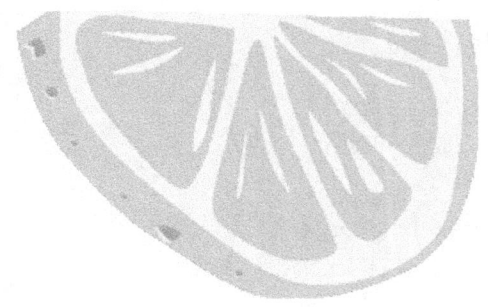

This fruit is a miraculous product known to kill cancer cells in the human body. It is 10,000 times stronger than Chemotherapy. It has a pleasant taste and does not produce the horrific effects.

As we know, the lemon/lime trees produce many varieties of fruit and can be eaten in different ways. Eat the pulp, squeeze the juice, and make pastries.

It has great effect on cysts, tumors and is a proven remedy against cancers of all types. Research reports show Lemon/Lime destroys malignant cells in 12 different types of cancers including colon, breasts, lung, prostate, and pancreatic.

Most astonishingly, this type of therapy only destroys the malignant cells and does not affect healthy cells of the body.

Reported by: The Institute of Health Services, Baltimore, Maryland..

BENEFITS OF SOME HEALING FOODS

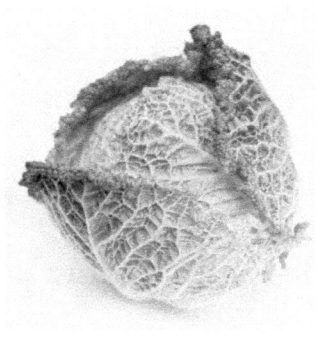

Cabbage:

- Stimulate digestion
- Activate detoxifying enzymes

Proven benefits: Stomach ulcers, constipation, headaches, skin care, eczema, arthritis, Digestive health, rheumatism, gout, weight loss.

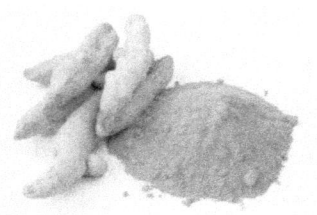

Turmeric (yellow ginger):

- Detoxifies the liver
- Flush out carcinogenic material

Proven benefits: Diabetes, hypertension, cholesterol, pain, slows the growth of cancer cells, Relief of arthritic pain prevents Alzheimer's disease.

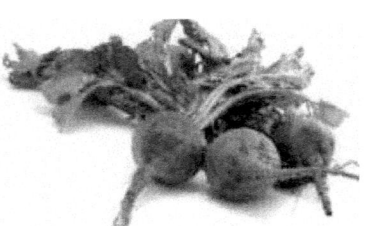

Beet root and leaves:

- Detoxifies and cleanse
- Creates acid/alkaline balance

Proven benefits: Decrease cancer causing material Anemia, arteriosclerosis, gout, blood pressure, cancer, kidney stones, gall bladder

Limes/lemons:

- High vitamin C
- Synthesizing toxic material

Proven benefits: Colds, flu, liver function, skin conditions; Drinking lime or lemon juice in the mornings help to boost liver function and excretory organs.

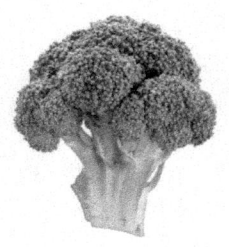

Broccoli:

- Enzyme production
- Flush out toxins

Proven benefits: liver health, natural enzymes, flushes out cancer cells, excretory organs.

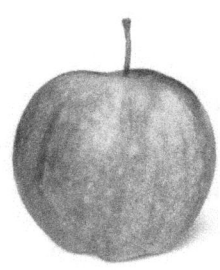

Apple:

- Contains pectin
- Liver function

Proven benefits: Contains the pectin enzyme, cleansing and detoxifying, improves digestive health; "An apple a day keeps the doctor away".

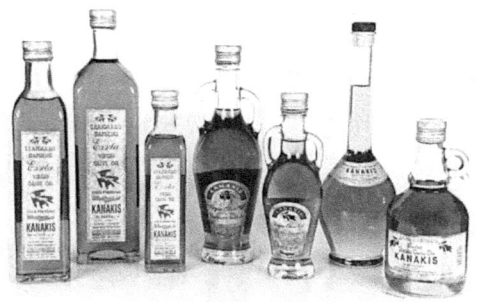

Natural cold-press oils (olive oil, coconut oil, flax seed oil, sesame seed oil) Provide lipid base to help the body decrease toxins, reduce toxic overload, promotes liver health.

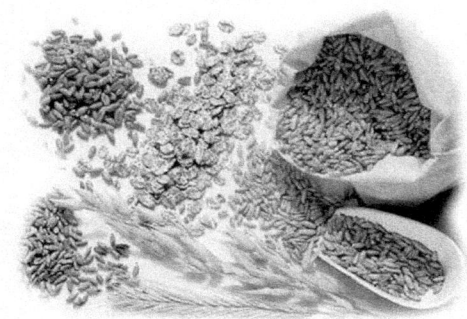

Whole Grains: (rye, wheat, brown rice etc.) Improve fat metabolization, rich in B vitamins

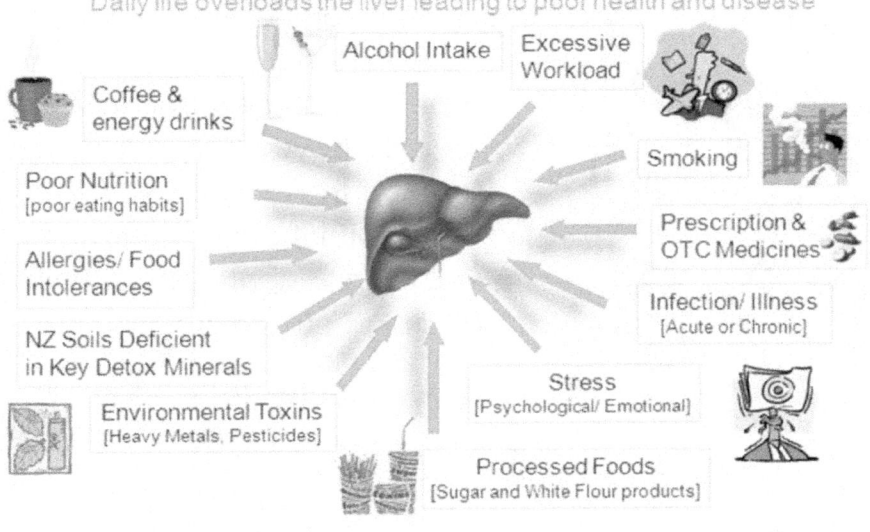

FLUSHING YOUR LIVER WITH OLIVE OIL & LEMON JUICE

Your liver is a vital organ; liver functions include filtering harmful substances, such as alcohol and caffeine, from your blood and storing vitamins and minerals. Liver and gallbladder cleanses are popular, yet controversial, methods of promoting liver health.

Flushing your liver with an olive oil and lemon juice tonic is a common cleansing technique. Although this flush has anecdotal support on alternative health websites, Michael Klaper, M.D., with the Institute of Nutrition Education and research, says that the olive oil and lemon juice cleanse is useless and, in some cases hazardous.

Consult your health care provider before attempting this liver flush.

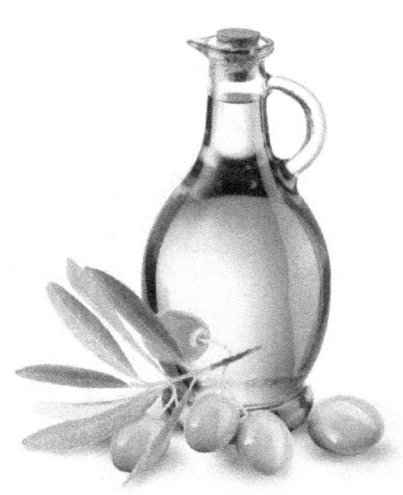

BENEFITS OF OLIVE OIL: Olive oil contains antioxidants that can protect you from strokes and heart attacks. Polyphenols, especially those found in virgin olive oil, have the ability to fight some of the conditions that come with the aging process, including weight gain, arthritis and high cholesterol.

Free radicals released as byproducts of natural metabolism and from some environmental pollutants damage cells and contribute to degenerative diseases. A scientific study published in the journal Molecular Nutrition & Food Research shows that the antioxidants in olive oil can help neutralize free radicals and limit or prevent their detrimental effects, thereby protecting red blood cells.

According to the Mayo Clinic, the monounsaturated fats in olive oil can help normalize your blood's ability to clot and benefit your insulin and blood sugar levels, along with fighting cholesterol. Because bile from the gallbladder is released when you eat food containing fat, drinking water with lemon juice and olive oil may help you expel gallstones.

FORGIVE and LET IT GO

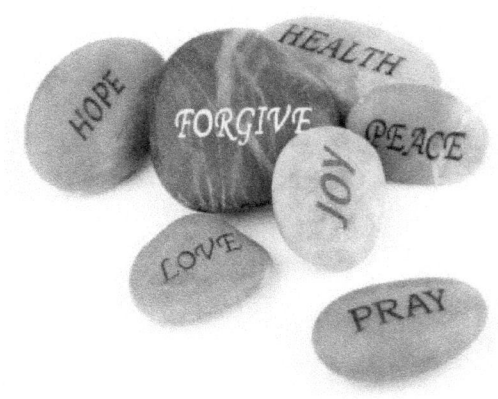

Hatred is an expression of fear and insecurity. Unforgiveness is the power that feeds hatred into the fabric of our personality and destroys our God-given power to succeed with our life goals.

When we forgive, we break the chain of Suffering; Once the chain is broken, the pain is removed Once the pain removed, the guilt flees, Once the guilt flees, our consciousness becomes free. Then we will forgive and forget past grudges. We will no longer hold on to them We basically, LET GO!!

FORGIVE for LOVE

FIVE SPIRITUAL PRINCIPLES
By the Teachers

Just for today, I give thanks for my many blessings,
Just for today, I will not worry
Just for today, I will not be angry
Today I will do my work honestly
Today I will be kind to my neighbor and every living thing.

THE LOTUS FLOWER The lotus flower Is one of the most ancient and deepest symbols of our planet. It grows in muddy water and rises above the surface to bloom with remarkable beauty. The flower loses at night and sinks underwater. Then rises and opens up again at dawn. This symbolizes purity of heart and mind.

Per Eastern belief, it represents long life, healthier, honor and good luck Though barely able to see the light through the muddy water, the new shoot strives upwards until eventually it bursts into the sunlight bringing the beauty of its delicate petals to the surface.

During their development, the plants filter and purify the body of the water in which they grow, changing the surroundings from murky to transparent and clean.

THE HOLISTIC INSTITUTE OF HEALING AND WELLNESS RESOURCE CENTER

THE HOLISTIC INSTITUTE OF HEALING, INC.
WELLNESS RESOURCE CENTER
BULLET TREE FALLS, CAYO, BELIZE, C.A

MISSION

THE MISSION OF THE HOLISTIC INSTITUTE OF HEALING and WELLNESS RESOURCES CENTER is to provide the highest level of preventive health care possible.

Our MISSION is accomplished by individuals completing a comprehensive self-assessment. Utilizing an Holistic approach participants are motivated to take the steps necessary to promote health and wellness.

GOALS:

- Wellness Support
- Health Education/Monitoring
- Client Empowerment
- Holistic Health Approach

Available for Health Education Classes: sessions focus on: Preventive Measures and Natural Healing Interventions Educational and training classes are individualized and conducted as one's own healing journey. All classes are held at the Healing and Wellness Resource Center. Material and supplies are available at a minimal cost.

To help you start your HEALING JOURNEY, we provide a thorough assessment, wellness intervention, recommendations, consultations and supportive care.

The Wellness Resource Center provides a peaceful place to help you transform and rejuvenate.

Steps to good health are encouraged through a change in attitude, and a change in behavior.

You are encouraged to make a serious commitment to develop and lead a healthy lifestyle. Experiences are provided to help you take control of your own health:

- JOURNALING
- WEIGHT LOSS - NUTRITIONAL COUNSELING
- EXERCISE
- MEDITATION
- VISUALIZATION
- THERAPEUTIC BATHING
- HERBS TO USE FOR HEALING
- REFLEXOLOGY
- CHAKRA BALANCING
- PREVENTATIVE HEALTH CARE INFORMATION
- DETOXIFICATION CLEANSING AND RESTORATION
- DIGESTIVE HEALTH/COLON CARE
- MENTAL - SPIRITUAL HEALTH COUNSELING
- BLOOD SUGAR LEVEL TESTING
- PRENATAL MONITORING
- BLOOD PRESSURE AND VITAL SIGN MONITORING
- GUIDED HEALING JOURNEYS

Calm your heart: Life always gives us what we need, when we need it!

WHO IS EUNICE M. CLARKE?

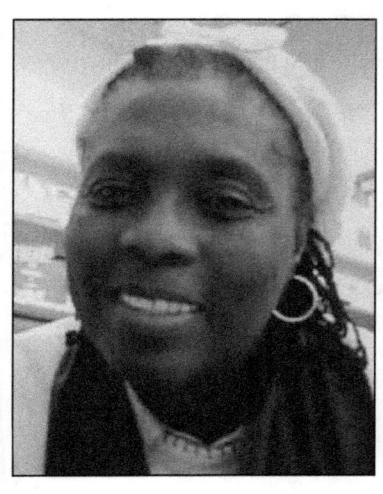

Rev. Eunice M. Clarke, Doctor of Christian Life /Family Counseling. A Holistic Nurse and Clinical Practitioner.

She is the founder and Director of the Holistic Institute of Healing: Wellness Resource Center.

As a qualified Holistic nurse and practitioner in both traditional and natural healing modalities, her experience spans over 25 years in the healthcare field.

Through clinical, administrative and educational aspects of acute, chronic and psychiatric arenas including educating clients on health and disease prevention, she is an experienced educator and advocate of nutritional healing and using nature's healing remedies where possible.

She is committed to the concept of wellness and allows consumer responsibility and self-care through training, education, and research.

Affirmation: Each day I AM Creating a new way of life

My Message: We are living in a very exciting and powerful time of life. On the deepest level of consciousness, a spiritual transformation is taking place. On a worldwide level, we are all being challenged to "Let Go" of our present way of life and create an entirely new one. In fact, we are in the process of releasing our "old and worn out "ways of living and create a NEW World in its place Surrender and allow the new style of life to manifest from the inside out.

HOLISTIC INSTITUTE OF HEALING (HEALING STATEMENTS)

Wellness is our natural state.

Disease is an impostor

The Divine dwells within you, and desires that you heal

Before you can heal others, you first have to heal yourself

Always leave some space within when you eat

Resisting change leads to illness.

Accepting change brings about peace

Illness begins in the stomach, and diet is the main remedy

Recovery a goal that you reach though a process

Health promotes spirituality, and spirituality promotes health

To heal the body, you must first heal the mind

Illness is not a punishment, but a stimulant to life

A cheerful expression brings joy to the heart, and good news, gives health to the bones

God doesn't create any illness, without also creating the remedy

Tranquility at home leads to health

Whatever is exposed to the light itself becomes light

Pain is the touchstone of spiritual progress

The root cause of all disease is a negative attitude about taking care of yourself

To heal illness, begin by restoring balance

The healthy person lives in harmony with nature

It's never too late to create a new body

Change your mind, change your life

By Dr. Geraldine Carter, Founder
Sacred Healing and Teaching Ministries,
Minnesota, USA

RECIPES FOR HEALTH

These recipes are only recommendations in times when the body feels sluggish and needs a boost.

Drink green tea for weight reduction and energy boost. Drink three to four cups daily.

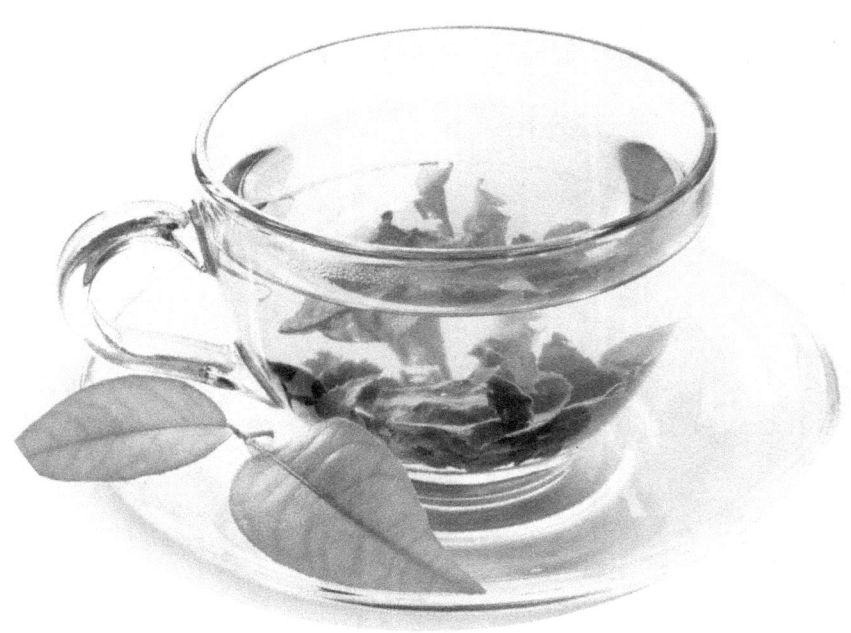

KALE SLAW AND RED CABBAGE

1 small grated red cabbage and 1 small green cabbage

1 apple

3 to 5 leaves fresh kale

2 medium size carrots, 3 radishes

Bean sprouts optional

Add Cilantro, Dill, Chives, Parsley, cayenne, as desired

Half teaspoon Sea Salt and 1 Tablespoon Vinaigrette

Soak grated cabbage, red and green, in water for 30 minutes then drain

Cut up apple into small chunks and toss in line and salt mixture

Add other ingredients

Store in covered bowl overnight and serve. Enjoy.

CITRUS GOLDEN POWER

YOUR FIRST MORNING DRINK

Ingredients

1 fresh squeezed lime or lemon juice or

may substitute 1 tablespoonful Bragg Apple Cider Vinegar

1 teaspoonful Turmeric Powder

1-4th teaspoonful ground black pepper

1 teaspoonful pure honey

8 ounces Warm water

Mix all ingredients and drink as a morning beverage. Use for 90 days.

CITRUS POWER

Ingredients

1 Squeezed Lime or Lemon Juice or

substitute 1 tablespoonful Bragg Apple Cider Vinegar

1 tablespoonful Olive Oil

1 tablespoonful Blackstrap Molasses

A pinch Cayenne Pepper

1 cupful warm water

Page 3. Recipes continue:

Directions_. Better to mix in a glass jar, shake about 20 times. Drink first thing in the mornings between 6am to 7am. Use for 30 days..

DETOX VEGGIE BROTH TO PROMOTE WEIGHT REDUCTION

Ingredients:

Carrots, Celery, Hichama, Beets optional,

Sweet potatoes, Daikon or Horseradish

Prepare vegetables into chunks,

Dulse, Cilantro, Thyme, Parsley, Fennel, 3 cloves Garlic, black pepper

Simmer for 2 to 3 hours, then add the juice of half squeezed lime,

Blend as desired. May use 2 or three times per week as desired.

Check the condition of your tongue, your skin, and body weight weekly. Record your progress in a journal.

Do not use fats and or carbohydrates combined with Detox veggie broth.

SUPER GREENS

Ingredients:

3 sticks Celery

1 handful Beet root greens, meaning leaves from Beet root.

1 handful Spinach

1 medium Carrot

1 medium Cucumber

1 piece White Ginger Root: size half your little finger.

1 Apple, 1 Lime Juice, 3 sprigs Parsley or Cilantro

10 ounces Water

Directions: wash vegetables thoroughly then soak in vinegar solution {half cupful vinegar to 1-pint water] May blend all ingredients in a Blender or use a Juicer. Juice all vegetables and fruit except the lime.

Squeeze lime juice separately and add to vegetable juice.

You may use this juice daily for 20 days to detoxify the body cells.

SOUP BLEND, LUNCH OR DINNER:

Ingredients:

3 cups ripened Tomatoes

1 cupful chopped Sweet Peppers

2 cups chopped Carrots

1 medium Red Onion

1 wedge Green Cabbage

2 cups yellow Pumpkin

2 sticks Celery

1 small Cucumber 1 Lime or Lemon juice

1 pinch Cayenne Pepper

1-4th teaspoon Yellow Ginger

1 teaspoonful Cumin

3 cloves Garlic

3 leaves Oregano leaves, Cilantro as desired

Directions: Wash vegetables thoroughly then soak for 5 minutes in vinegar solution: half cup vinegar to one-pint water. Then chop and dice tomatoes, sweet peppers, carrots, red onions, cabbage, celery, cucumber. Mix in a large bowl and divide in half into two separate bowls. To bowl # 1 add grated yellow pumpkin, cayenne, yellow ginger, chopped garlic and oregano. Cook for 10 minutes then allow to cool, then blend the cooked ingredients to puree. To bowl #2 add

pureed vegetables, salt and lime juice to taste. Cover and allow to set over night in the refrigerator. Use for lunch or dinner meal.

Alkalize and Hydrate with Green Juice

Ingredients:

Coconut water and meat

3 slices Pineapple and 1 wedge Watermelon

2 Cucumbers

1 bunch Parsley, Cilantro, lime juice, thumb size ginger

Wash and blend all ingredients together. May add ice cubes on a hot day.

Benefits: Delicious, energizing, hydrating and rebalancing electrolytes. Balances Blood Sugar. Alleviates constipation. This is a GI Tract cleanser, freshens the breath, energizes the body and mind.

    ENJOY.......

SOME HEALTHFUL BENEFITS OF ALOE VERA:

Our ancestors called it the MEDICINE PLANT because it healed all ails. Every home relied on its healing benefits and its extracts as medicine for every member of the family…Many researchers of today are unearthing more and more healthful benefits of this ancient plant.

Many skin remedies.

Cooling and repairing sunburn skin

Hydrates skin cells

Protects the body from stress

Supports the immune system

Strengthens gums and promotes strong and healthy teeth

Heals the Intestines and lubricates the digestive tract

Lowers high cholesterol levels

Stabilizes blood sugar levels

Prevents kidney stones formation

Reduces high blood pressure

Detoxifies the body

Soothes arthritis pain

Prevents and treats Candida Infections.

Helps to heal insect stings, blisters, allergic reactions, burns, eczema, psoriasis, inflammation hard to heal wounds.

Boosts cardiovascular performance and physical endurance.

Reference: Rawforbeauty.com

The Holistic Institute of Healing and Wellness Resource Center Volunteer Opportunities

Opportunities for Students
Spring Break Program –
Time: Second Week of March, 7 to 9 days

Target Projects:
- Create garden plots (raised beds)
- Build thatch cabana
- Harvest and process herbs
- Learn about herbal medicine
- Sample local popular herbal teas and drinks around the village
- Learn raw and cooked food prep of local fruits and vegetables
- Independently create healthy dish for group potluck

Optional Additions:
- Develop, organize, and run a one-week reading program (ages 9 -11; 1 hour per day)
- Receive massage therapy, steam bath, herbal bath, or colonic irrigation
- Attend local yoga or tai chi classes
- Visit Mayan Ruins
- Visit Spanish Lookout

Cost: Varies by year. Email essai963c@yahoo.com to inquire.

What's Included:

Shared housing, three meals per day, project materials, clean water, access to Wi-Fi, and airport pickup/drop-off

Summer Break Program –
Time: May through August

First Session: June 1 – June 14
Second Session: June 19 – June 30
Third Session: July 6 – July 15

Target Projects:
- Design S.M.A.R.T Program
- Execute S.M.A.R.T Program
- Develop Program Projects

Description of the S.M.A.R.T. Program:
The program is designed to help youth maintain their study skills in basic Reading and Mathematics. There will be games for reinforcing Math and Reading skills. The program will be enjoyable for both students and parents. It will provide activities that encourage leadership, community pride with emphasis on appreciation for the environment.

Example: gardening, nutrition, personal hygiene, including hand washing, healthy eating, food Preservation by dehydrating and freezing; linking learning to real life experience.

There will be opportunity for the 12 to 13-year-old students to take part in the volunteerism and mentoring the younger age groups. This will encourage development of leadership, self-esteem building, and self-discipline. All participants in the SMART Program will learn how to identify and utilize natural resources which are found in Belize.

Some other activities:
- Two day trips to Natural Resource Parks
- Graduation activities

Cost: Varies by year. Email essai963c@yahoo.com to inquire.

What's included:
Shared housing, three meals per day, project materials, clean water, access to Wi-Fi, and airport pickup/drop-off

Winter Break Program –
Time: December 15 – December 22 (7 days), December 26 – January 8 (13 days), or December 15 – January 8 (24 days)

Target Projects:
- Create garden plots (raised beds)
- Build thatch cabana
- Harvest and process herbs
- Learn about herbal medicine
- Sample local popular herbal teas and drinks around the village
- Learn raw and cooked food prep of local fruits and vegetables
- Independently create healthy dish for group potluck

Optional Additions:
- Develop, organize, and run a one-week reading program (ages 9 -11; 1 hour per day)
- Develop, organize, and run reading competition for local children
- Develop, organize, and run Spelling Bee for local children
- Receive massage therapy, steam bath, herbal bath, or colonic irrigation
- Attend local yoga or tai chi classes
- Visit Mayan Ruins
- Visit Spanish Lookout

Cost: Varies by year. Email essai963c@yahoo.com to inquire.

What's included:

Shared housing, three meals per day, project materials, clean water, access to Wi-Fi, and airport pickup/drop-off

Rules for All Yaya's Global Volunteers:

- No alcohol or tobacco
- No drugs on or off premises
- Must have travel/health insurance
- No medical or health disabilities (We are not equipped to handle disabilities at this time – our apologies.)
- Volunteer/work – 4 to 6 hours a day
- Free time daily for self-enhancement

www.ingramcontent.com/pod-product-compliance
Lightning Source LLC
Chambersburg PA
CBHW070106210526
45170CB00013B/765